NEW ANTI-INFLAMMATORY DIET COOKBOOK
—FOR—
BEGINNERS

ESSENTIAL MEALS WITH POWERS TO HEAL... CHOSEN DELICIOUS EASY RECIPES TO REDUCE INFLAMMATION...

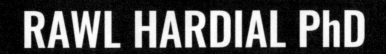

RAWL HARDIAL PhD

New Anti-Inflammatory Diet Cookbook for Beginners

Essential Meals with Powers to Heal…

Chosen Delicious Easy Recipes to Reduce Inflammation…

Author: Dr Rawl Hardial

Thank you for choosing this book. As much as I do, I hope you enjoy all the exciting recipes within this book to a healthier happier pain free life….

Copyright © 2020 by Rawl Hardial PhD. All rights reserved.

This new anti-inflammatory diet cook book for beginners contains advice and information relating to health care. It is not intended to replace medical advice and should be used to supplement rather than replace regular care by your doctor. It is recommended that you seek your doctor's advice before starting any medical program or treatment. All efforts have been made to assure the accuracy of the information contained in this book as of the date of publication. The author disclaims liability for any medical outcome that may occur as a result of applying the methods suggested in this book.

No part of this new anti-inflammatory diet cook book for beginners may be reproduced in any form or by any electronic or mechanical means. This includes information storage and retrieval systems, without written permission from the author, except for the use of brief quotations in a book review.

TABLE OF CONTENTS

Introduction, "Why You Might Need the New Anti-Inflammatory Diet Cookbook For Beginners" 1

    What is Inflammation? 1

    Anti-Inflammatory Diet 1

    Foods to Eat 2

    Other Helpful Tips 2

Chapter One: - Foods That Cause Inflammation 3

    Sugar 3

    TRANS FAT 3

    Carbohydrates 4

    Red Meat 4

    Alcohol 5

    Bottom line 5

Chapter Two: - Anti-Inflammatory healthy Breakfast Recipes 6

    Baked rice porridge recipe with fruit 6

    Ingredients 6

    Instructions 7

    Herb-Baked Eggs 8

    Ingredients 8

    Instruction 8

    Coffee and Mint Yogurt Parfait 9

    Ingredients 9

    Instructions 9

    Cinnamon Granola Crunchy 10

    Ingredients 10

Instructions 10

Pineapple Anti-Inflammatory Smoothie 12

Ingredients 12

Instructions 13

Pecan Banana Bread and Oats Recipe 14

Ingredients 14

Yogurt Parfait with Raspberries and Chia Seeds 16

Ingredients 16

Instructions 16

Anytime Breakfast Bowl 17

INGREDIENTS 17

Instructions 18

Greek Yogurt Smoothie Recipe 19

Ingredients 19

Instructions 19

Cacao Berry Smoothie 20

Ingredients 20

Instructions 20

Avocado Toast with Egg 21

Ingredients 21

Instructions 21

Chia Quinoa Porridge 22

Ingredients 22

Ingredients 22

Vanilla Turmeric Orange Juice 23

Ingredients 23

Instructions 23

No-Bake Turmeric Protein Donuts 24

Ingredients 24

Instructions 24

Golden Milk Chia Seed Pudding 26

Ingredients 26

Instructions 27

Chapter Three: - Anti-Inflammatory Lunch Recipes 28

Smashed Chickpea Avocado Salad Sandwich with Cranberries + Lemon 28

Ingredients 28

Instructions 29

Walnut-Rosemary Crusted Salmon 30

Ingredients 30

Instructions 31

Artichoke ricotta flatbread 32

INGREDIENTS 32

Instructions 33

Miso-Maple Salmon 34

Ingredients 34

Instructions 34

Broccoli & Cauliflower Salad 36

Ingredients 36

Instructions 36

Roasted Beet Hummus 38

Ingredients 38

Instructions 38

Five-Spice Bacon salad WITH PEACH, Raspberry & Watercress 39

Ingredients 39

Instruction 40

Beet & Goat Cheese Tartines 41

Ingredients 41

Instruction 41

Turmeric Rice Bowl with Garam Masala Root Vegetables & Chickpeas 43

Ingredients 43

Instructions 44

Roasted Root Veggies & Greens over Spiced Lentils 45

Ingredients 45

Instructions 46

Fish Tacos with Broccoli Slaw and Cumin Sour Cream 47

Ingredients 47

Instructions 48

Whole-Grain Cinnamon French Toast With Broiled Grapes 49

Ingredients 49

Instructions 50

Chapter Four: - Dinner Recipes 51

Chickpea and Vegetable Coconut Curry 51

Ingredients 51

Instructions 52

White Turkey Chili with Avocado 53

Ingredients 53

Instructions 53

Chicken and Snap Pea Stir-Fry 55

Ingredients 55

Instructions 56

Greek Turkey Burgers 57

Ingredients 57

Dijon Salmon with Green Bean Pilaf 59

Ingredients 59

Instructions 60

Ginger Meatball Ramen with Greens and Scallions 61

Ingredients 61

For serving 62

Soy-Glazed Salmon Sandwiches with Watercress 63

Ingredients 63

Instructions 64

Mole-Spiced Black Bean and Quinoa Bowl 65

Ingredients 65

Instructions 66

Vegan Green Edamame Spinach Hummus Pesto 67

Ingredients 67

Instructions 68

Vegan Deep Dish Falafel Pizza 69

Ingredients 69

Instructions 70

Chapter Five: - Snack Recipes 71

TURMERIC BARS 71

Ingredients 71

Instructions 72

Turmeric Gummies 73

Ingredients 73

Instructions 73

Spicy Tuna Rolls 74

- Ingredients 74
- Instructions 74
- Spicy Kale Chips 75
- Ingredients 75
- Instructions 75
- Peasy Ginger Date Bars 76
- Ingredients 76
- Instructions 76
- Turmeric Coconut Flour Muffins Recipe 77
- Ingredients 77
- Instructions 77

Chapter Six: - Conclusion, Benefits of Anti-Inflammatory diet 79

Authors Final thought 80

Introduction, "Why You Might Need the New Anti-Inflammatory Diet Cookbook For Beginners"

What is Inflammation?

Inflammation is a means of defending the body from infection, illness, or injury. The immune system identifies and initiates the healing process through to the damaged cells, irritants, and pathogens. A biological response occurs when something harmful or unpleasant happens to a part of our body. The biological response is to try to eliminate the intruder.

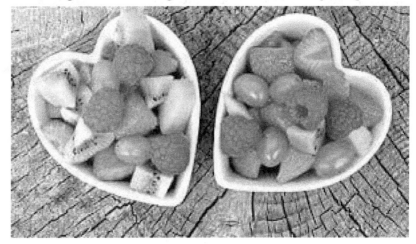

Your body raises white blood cells, immune cells, and cytokines that help battle infection during inflammatory reactions.

Anti-Inflammatory Diet

An anti-inflammatory diet is commonly considered safe, and it can help the risk of having other complications even if it doesn't help with your disease. However, researchers are still finding out how inflammation can affect what we eat. So far, eating a variety of nutritious foods tends to help minimize inflammation in the body.

What we eat will help avoid chronic inflammation and keep it under control. Focus your diet on nutrient-rich whole foods containing antioxidants and avoid refined items.

Antioxidants function by reducing free radical rates. These reactive molecules are formed as a normal part of our metabolism, but if they are not regulated, they can lead to inflammation.

Your anti-inflammatory diet will maintain a balanced protein, carbs, and fat balance at every meal. Make sure you do fulfill the vitamin, mineral, food, and water requirements of your body. Inflammation can be improved by healthy fats, such as monounsaturated fats and omega-3 fatty acids.

In general, the anti-inflammatory diet and lifestyle is an effective way of reducing pain rates. Importantly, this pain control strategy is free of adverse side effects. Unpleasant side effects of certain medicines are no longer a concern.

Foods to Eat

An anti-inflammatory diet is commonly considered to be safe, so it will reduce your risk of having other issues even if it does not benefit your condition. On the one side, it helps protect the body from infection and injury. On the other side, inflammatory diets can lead to weight gain and illness. This risk can be made much greater by unhealthy foods and low levels of activity.

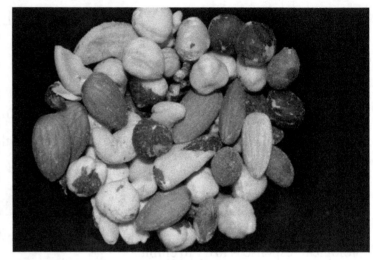

However, much research indicates that certain foods may be able to combat inflammation. Below are the lists of foods that are anti-inflammatory.

- **Vegetables:** cauliflower, cabbage, Brussels sprouts, Broccoli, kale,
- **Fruit:** cherries, strawberries, blueberries, raspberries, blackberries, grapes
- **High-fat fruits:** olives and Avocados
- **Healthy fats:** Extra virgin olive oil and coconut oil
- **Fatty fish:** anchovies, herring, mackerel, sardines, Salmon,
- **Nuts:** Almonds
- **Peppers:** chili peppers, Bell peppers
- **Chocolate:** cocoa and Dark chocolate
- **Spices:** fenugreek, Turmeric, cinnamon, etc
- **Tea:** Green tea

Other Helpful Tips

Supplements: Some supplements that reduce inflammation are fish oil and curcumin.

Daily exercise: Exercise will reduce the risk of chronic disease and inflammatory markers

Sleep: Studies found that a bad night's sleep causes inflammation. You can enhance the benefits of your anti-inflammatory diet by taking some supplements and ensuring you get enough workouts and sleep.

Chapter One: - Foods That Cause Inflammation

The body's normal processes to increase blood flow where there is pain and causing redness due to the increased blood supply are called Inflammation. It helps to battle infections or toxins in an attempt to heal them. This is a normal response when occasionally occurring, called acute inflammation think of a bruise or swollen ankle that lasts just a few days.

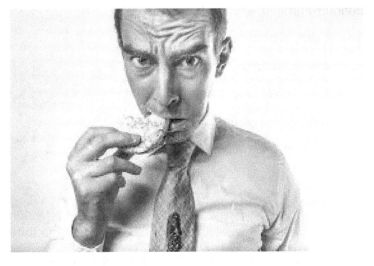

Yet, chronic symptoms can lead to severe health issues such as heart disease, cancer, recurrent lower respiratory infection, asthma, Alzheimer's disease, psoriasis and stroke.

An inflammatory diet is one of the most significant natural forms in which inflammation can be regulated. Below are several foods that may lead to or intensify the inflammation.

Sugar

Nutrition experts Frances Largeman-Roth, RDN, author of Eating in Colour, claim the release of cytokines can increase chronic inflammation, and foods such as packaged granola bars, cereals, and fancy coffee drinks can increase chronic inflammation by releasing cytokines and can also increase blood pressure.

Excessive high-fructose corn syrup and other sugar may also raise the risk of type 2 diabetes, insulin resistance, and cancer, adds Orgain's founder and CEO Andrew Abraham, MD.

We should not equate these foods with natural sugars such as fruits, vegetables, whole grains, and milk, while it is not necessary to eliminate all extra sugars from our diets, we can tolerate our everyday intake. "Start your morning coffee with fewer sweeteners and eventually hit nil," advises Largeman-Roth.

Trans Fat

Tran's fat (also called trans-unsaturated fat) is the 'bad' form of dietary fat. Tran's fat intake is directly related to inflammation, which raises the risk of chronic conditions like diabetes and heart disease. Tran's fat also increases the body's low-density lipoprotein (LDL) cholesterol (the "bad" type) and decreases its high-density lipoprotein (HDL) cholesterol (the "healthy or good" type). Most fast-food products, such as

French fries and other fried foods, as well as candy and other commonly recognized unhealthy foods, contain transfat.

However, not all fats are equal. Harvard Health Publishing defines Tran's fat as the worst type, while saturated fat falls somewhere in the middle. The "healthy" fats are the monounsaturated and polyunsaturated fats. A diet containing some saturated, monounsaturated, and polyunsaturated fats can have the most benefits. Saturated fat is present in foods like red meat, cheese, whole milk, and other processed foods. Although not considered harmful as the dreaded 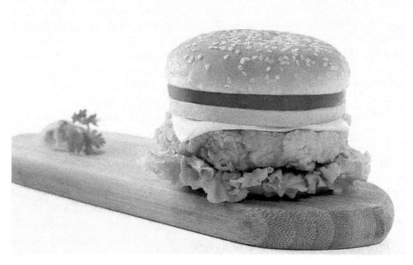 Tran's fat, saturated fat has been linked to inflammation and other killer diseases and as a result should only be eaten in moderation. Better fats are found in olive oil, almond, canola, safflower, and sunflower; most nuts; and avocados. Such foods should be eaten in moderation because too much may have harmful effects. So moderation is the key!

CARBOHYDRATES

Processed carbohydrates are "simple carbs/ refined carbs" and have little to no nutritional benefit. The body digests these carbohydrates rapidly, and because of their high glycemic index, the use of simple carbohydrates raises the blood sugar levels. Those carbohydrates entered as sugars into the bloodstream. Eating processed carbohydrates can quickly spike your insulin levels. After consuming, you quickly feel hungry again, as well as boost your cravings for more sweet carbohydrates.

"Natural" carbohydrates are foods such as wheat and rice, but when made into food items like pizza dough, bread, donut, specific candy, cereals, and other snacks are usually defined as processed carbohydrates.

RED MEAT

"Usually, meat consists of high arachidonic acid levels as well as saturated fat, which contributes to inflammation," Dr. Abraham said.

The doctor advises us that consuming more vegetarian food is one easy and general form of combating inflammation. Plant proteins typically have much less fat, particularly saturated fat. "Plant-based diets containing lots of leafy greens as well as anti-inflammatory foods influence the body. This, on the other side, lowers the likelihood of cancer and, above all, all who consume more plant-based options in their diet simply feel much better. Studies show they have better skin, and general overall health.

ALCOHOL

In the "Whole Body Cure", Kirshner states that, in addition to increasing inflammation, daily alcohol intake may interact with bacterial bacteria, change the structure and function of the brain, raise blood pressure and increase the risk of stroke, cardiac disease, and type 2 diabetes.

BOTTOM LINE

The bottom line: check for labels before buying and remove hydrogenated fats, added sugar, and processed carbohydrates. Consume a diet full of vegetables and fruits, spices and herbs, olive oil, healthy fish, and nuts.

Chapter Two: - Anti-Inflammatory healthy Breakfast Recipes

Baked rice porridge recipe with fruit

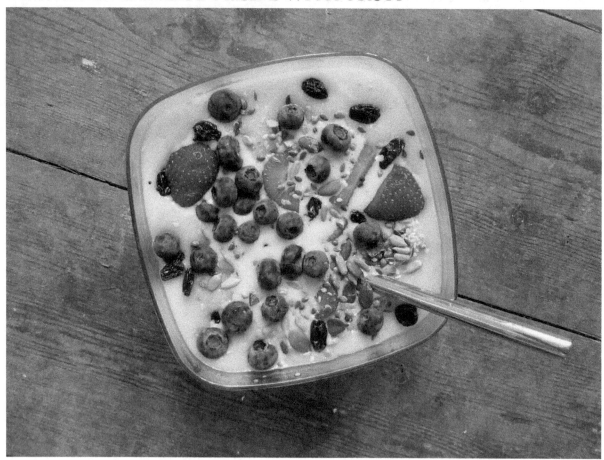

Ingredients

- Brown rice ½ cups
- Pure vanilla extract ½ teaspoon
- Cinnamon to taste
- Pure maple syrup two tablespoons
- Sliced fruit, cherries, plums, pears, berries,
- Optional
- Salt if needed or desired

INSTRUCTIONS

- Preheat the oven to 400 ° C.
- Add or place the water and rice in a pot over medium-high heat. Take the vanilla and cinnamon extract to a simmer, then whisk. Cook for about 10-15 minutes until tender (or for packing instructions when using a variety of rice that takes longer to cook).
- Place the rice in two heat-safe bowls or containers. Top each bowl with a fruit of your choice and the tablespoon of maple syrup. Add salt if desired.
- Cook or Bake for about 10 to 15 minutes before the maple syrup bursts, and the fruit begins to caramelize. Serve right away

Herb-Baked Eggs

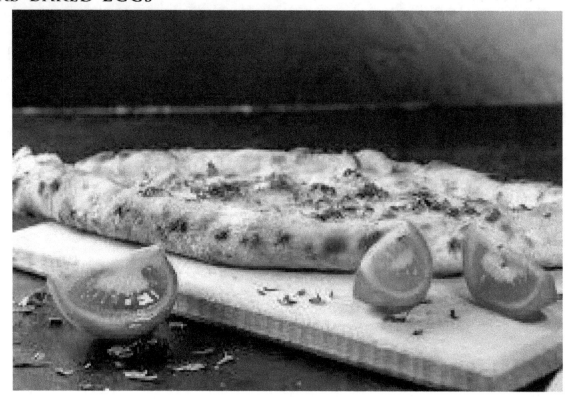

Ingredients
- Melted butter one teaspoon
- Milk 1 tablespoon
- Eggs 2
- Sprinkle, dried dill, dried parsley, dried oregano, dried thyme, and garlic powder,

Instruction
- Adjust your oven "Broil" mode on low
- Cover or coat the bottom of a small baking dish with milk and butter.
- Crack the eggs over the butter and milk mixture. Sprinkle with garlic and herbs.
- Cook or Bake for 5-6 minutes before the eggs are cooked to your satisfaction.

Coffee and Mint Yogurt Parfait

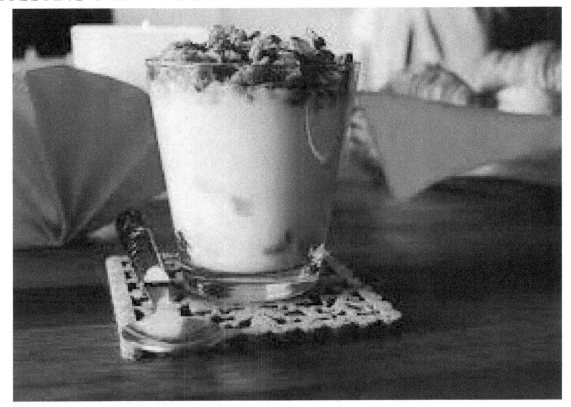

Ingredients
- Plain yogurt ½ cups
- Brewed coffee 2 teaspoons
- Pecans chopped ¼ cup

Optional
- Peppermint 3-4 drops

For garnish
- Fresh mint and coffee granules

Instructions
- In a small bowl mix yogurt, coffee, and stevia
- Layer the yogurt with the pecan a small glass
- Garnish with fresh mint and coffee granules

Cinnamon Granola Crunchy

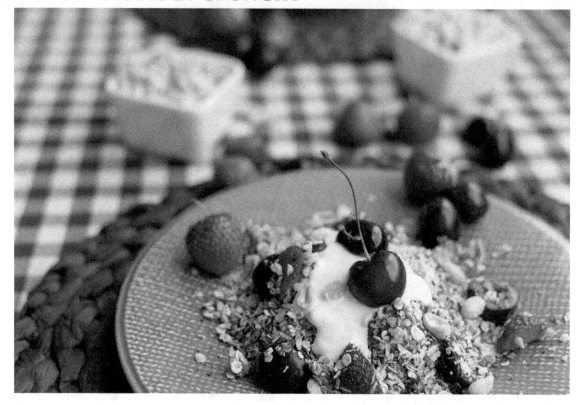

Ingredients

- Old-fashioned rolled oats 2 cups
- Unsweetened shredded coconut ¼ cup
- Pumpkin seeds 2 tablespoons
- Ground cinnamon ½ teaspoon
- Ground cloves ¼ teaspoon
- Ground nutmeg ¼ teaspoon
- Honey ¼ cup
- Melted, unsalted butter 4 tablespoons
- Raisins ¼ cup
- Dried apricots chopped ¼ cup
- Dried cranberries ¼ cup

Instructions

- Preheat the oven to 300 degrees Celsius.
- Fill or line the baking sheet with parchment paper

- Add the oats, coconuts, walnuts, seeds, and spices in a large mixing bowl and set aside.
- Add the honey and the melted butter in a separate bowl, and then pour over the oat mixture. Until stir Well,
- Place the mix of the oat on the baking sheet. Bake for about 25 minutes until it looks brown. Turn the oven off and set aside until cool.
- Crush the granola into the dried fruit when it cools and mixes.

Pineapple Anti-Inflammatory Smoothie

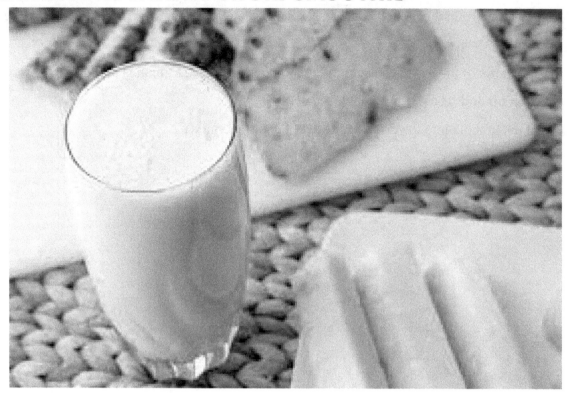

Ingredients

- Cooled green tea brewed and 1 cup
- Kale or spinach 2 cups
- Pineapple chunks frozen 1 cup
- Cucumber, peeled and cut into large chunks ⅔ cup
- Mango chunks frozen ½ cup
- Medium banana, peeled ½
- Fresh ginger peeled and cut from stalk ½ tsp
- Ground turmeric ¼ tsp
- Mint leaves- rough chopped 3
- Protein powder 1 scoop
- Chia seeds 1 Tbsp
- Ice cubes 4-5

INSTRUCTIONS

- Combine all, except chia seeds, in a high-speed blender.
- After the blending phase is completed, add chia seeds so that they do not bind to the blender container.
- Add the ice cubes if you want a smoother smoothie and blend until the desired consistency is reached.

Pecan Banana Bread and Oats Recipe

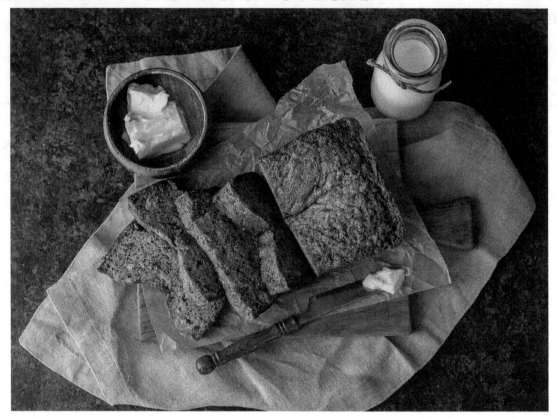

Ingredients

- Old-fashioned rolled oats 1 cup
- Milk 1 1/2
- Ripe bananas, mashed 2
- Greek yogurt plain 1/4 cup
- Coconut flakes unsweetened, toasted
- Honey 2 Tbsp
- Chia seeds 1 Tbsp
- Vanilla extracts 2 tsp
- Flaked sea salt 1/4 tsp

For serving

- Pomegranate seeds, honey, fig halves, roasted pecans, and Banana slices,
- Ingredients
- in a small bowl Stir the oats, Greek yogurt; uncooked coconut flakes; honey; chia seeds; vanilla extract, sea salt, milk, and bananas, until well combined

- Divide the mixture into two glass jars or bowls. Cover and cool for at least 6 hours or overnight.

For Topping
- Add banana slices, honey, roasted pecans, and fig halves Pomegranate seeds

Yogurt Parfait with Raspberries and Chia Seeds

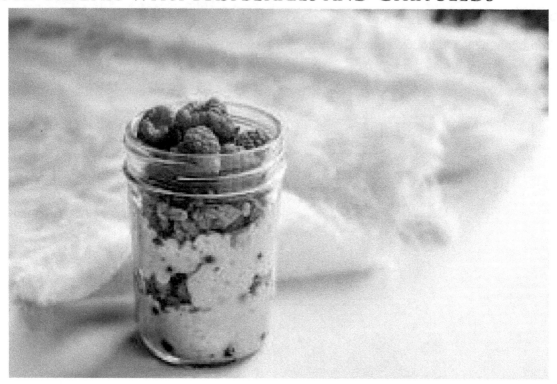

Ingredients
- Raspberries fresh ½ cup
- Chia seeds 2 tablespoons
- Maple syrup 1 teaspoon
- Cinnamon to taste
- Plain yogurt 16-ounces
- Fresh fruit, strawberries, nectarines, sliced blackberries

Instructions
- Put the raspberries in a small mixing pot or bowl or glass jar. Mash the berries on the back of the fork until it looks like Jam.
- In a small bowl, add honey, Chia seeds, and cinnamon and mash until fully combine then set aside.
- Place the yogurt coating at the bottom of a medium-sized glass or bowl.
- Add a new layer of the chia raspberry mixture for topping. Then add a layer of yogurt. Garnish with freshly cut fruit and a drizzle of extra maple syrup, if necessary.

Anytime Breakfast Bowl

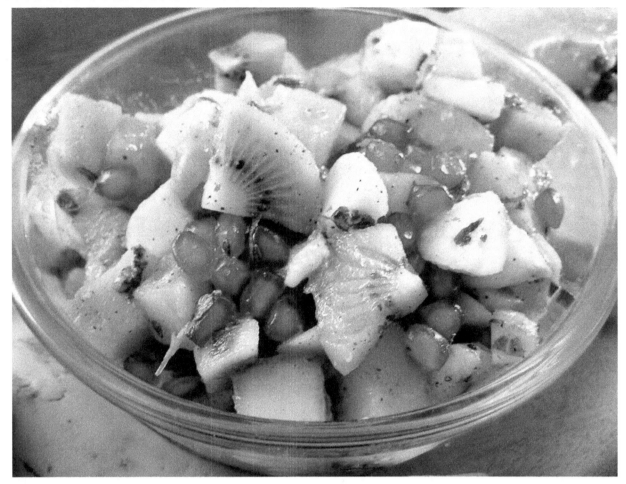

INGREDIENTS

- Grains such as buckwheat, amaranth, or quinoa 1 cup
- Coconut water or nut milk 2½ cups
- Cinnamon stick 1
- Whole cloves 2
- **Fresh Fruit:** blackberries, persimmons, cranberries, apples, pears, kiwi, mango

Optional

- Maple syrup
- Star anise pod 1

Instructions

- In a saucepan, add spices, grain, and coconut water or nut milk and bring to a boil. Cook for about 25-35 minutes until the grains are soft or tender. Take all the herbs out of the saucepan.
- Serve with the favorite berries or fruits and a drizzle of maple syrup, if necessary.

Greek Yogurt Smoothie Recipe

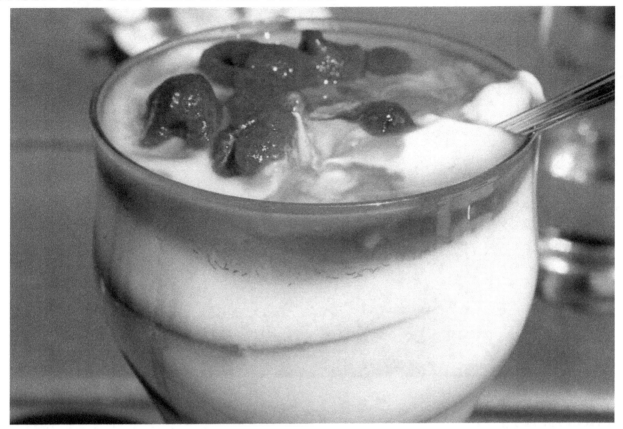

Ingredients

- Nut milk of choice, such as cashew milk, almond milk, 1- cup
- Greek yogurt plain ½ cups
- Baby spinach packed ¼ cup
- Blueberries frozen or fresh ¼ cup
- Nut butter of choice such as peanut butter, almond butter 1 tablespoon
- Ice cubes 3-4

For topping:

- Bee pollen or pistachios, cardamom, or a pinch of ground cinnamon

Instructions

- In a medium, the blender adds all ingredients and blends well until smooth.
- Serve

Cacao Berry Smoothie

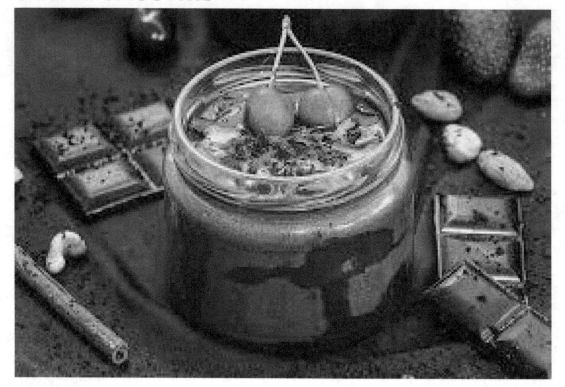

Ingredients

- Coconut, milk or Almond 1-cup
- Filtered water 1/2 cup
- Baby spinach fresh1 cup
- Raspberries fresh or frozen1 cup
- Banana 1
- Cacao powder 3 tablespoons
- Maple syrup or honey 1 tablespoon
- Ice 2-3 cubes

Optional

- Cacao nibs

Instructions

- Add all ingredients in a medium blender and blend well until liquefied.
- Fill or top with cacao nibs if desired.
- Serve and Enjoy

Avocado Toast with Egg

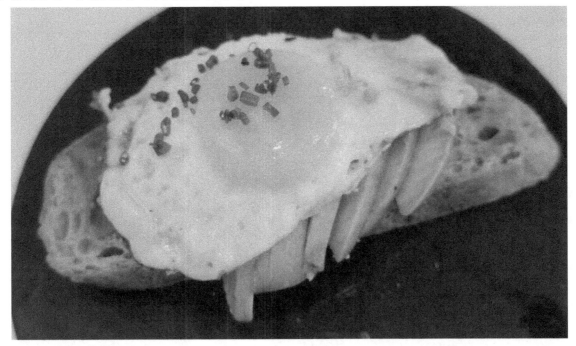

Ingredients

- Toasted, gluten-free bread 1 slice
- Oil 1½ tsp
- Avocado ½
- Spinach "Handful"
- Egg, poached or scrambled 1
- Red pepper to taste

Instructions

- Add oil and toast gluten-free bread
- Place the avocado over the toast. Place the spinach "fresh" on top of the avocado and top with scrambled egg or poached and sprinkle with the red pepper
- Repeat the same steps with second toast and serve as a sandwich

Chia Quinoa Porridge

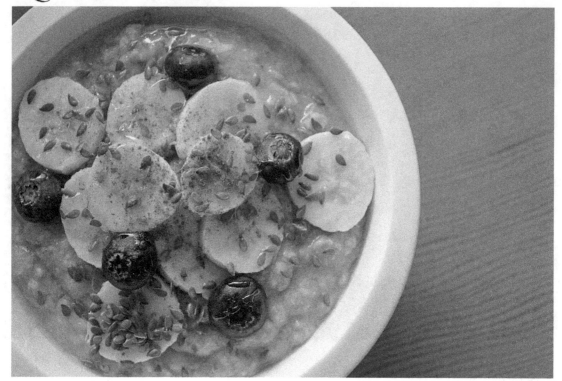

Ingredients

- Cashew milk thick 1 cup
- Quinoa cooked 2 cups
- Organic blueberries fresh 1 cup
- Walnuts toasted ¼ cup
- Ground cinnamon ½ tsp
- Honey "raw" 2 tsp
- Chia seeds Tbsp

Ingredients

- Mix the Cashew milk and Quinoa milk in a small saucepan with low, medium heat and steam slowly.
- Add and stir the blueberries, cinnamon, and walnuts until all are evenly cooked, then away from heat and set aside and Add honey and wait until stir completely and fill up the chia seeds.
- Topped with raw cacao nibs, sliced banana and serve.

Vanilla Turmeric Orange Juice

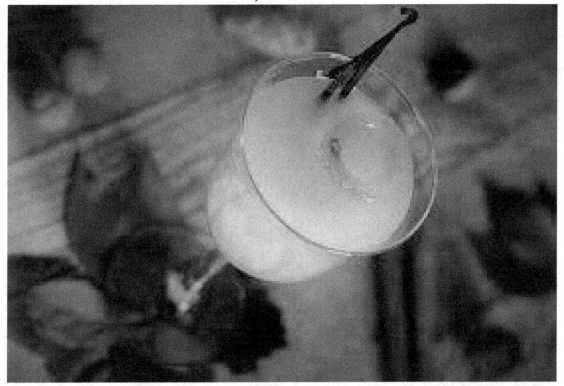

Ingredients
- Peeled oranges, quartered 3
- Almond milk unsweetened 1 cup
- Vanilla extracts 1tsp
- Cinnamon ½ tsp
- Turmeric ¼ turmeric
- Pepper to taste

Instructions
- Add all ingredients in a blender and blend well until smooth.
- Serve

No-Bake Turmeric Protein Donuts

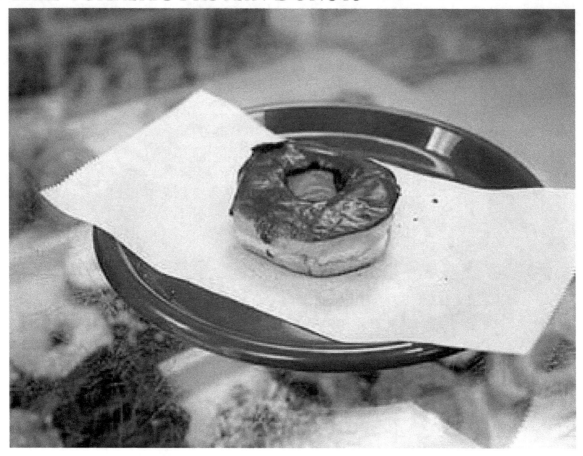

Ingredients

- Cashews raw 1½ cups
- Dates pitted Medjool ½ cup 7 pieces
- Vanilla protein powder 1 tsp
- Coconut shredded ¼ cup
- Maple syrup 2tsp
- Vanilla essence ¼ tsp
- Turmeric powder 1 tsp

For topping

- Chocolate dark ¼ cup

Instructions

- Combine all ingredients except chocolate and process in a food processor until the smooth and sticky cookie dough is created.

- Roll and Shape batter to 8 balls, then push the silicone donut mold firmly.
- Cover mold with plastic or lid and put it in the freezer for 30 minutes.
- For the chocolate topping
- Add a cup of water in a small boil and bring it to boil.
- Place a small saucepan over the bowl and add the chocolate into the bowl. Stir softly until the chocolate has melted.
- Remove donuts from mold and drizzle with chocolate and store into the fridge and serve

Golden Milk Chia Seed Pudding

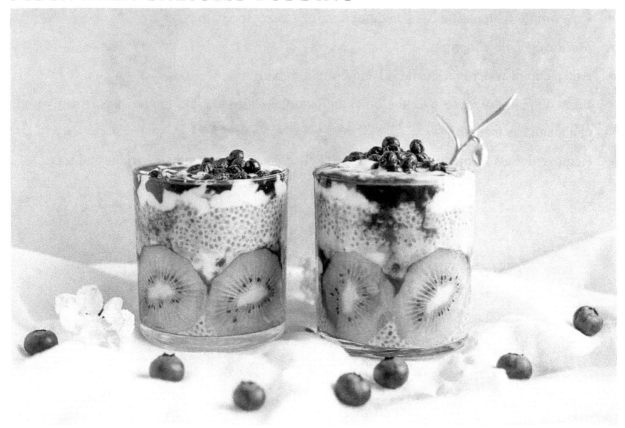

Ingredients

- Coconut milk full-fat 4 cups
- Honey 3tsp
- Vanilla extracts 1 tsp
- Turmeric ground 1tsp
- Cinnamon ground 1 tsp
- Ginger ground 1 tsp
- Chia seeds ½ cup
- For topping
- Coconut yogurt ¾ cup

For garnishing

- Fresh mixed berries 1 cup
- Toasted coconut chips ¼ cup

Instructions

- Add honey, vanilla extract, turmeric, cinnamon ground ginger, and coconut milk in a large mixing bowl and mix well until looks like a vibrant yellow liquid.
- Add chia seeds in this liquid and then mix well and set aside for 4-10 minutes.
- Cover the bowl with lid and let it cool in the fridge for at least 7-8 hours or until chia seeds look like a plump and give the mixture a thick pudding consistency.
- In a four glass add chia seed pudding evenly then top with coconut yogurt and garnish with toasted coconut chips and berries

Chapter Three: - Anti-Inflammatory Lunch Recipes

Smashed Chickpea Avocado Salad Sandwich with Cranberries + Lemon

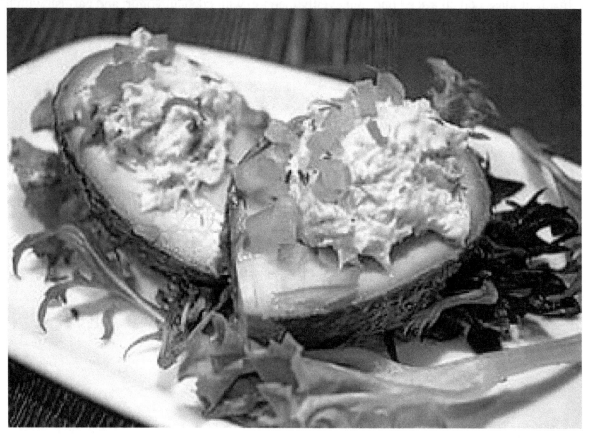

Ingredients
- Chickpeas drained and rinsed 1 - 15 oz can
- Avocado ripe large 1
- Lemon juice squeezed 2 teaspoon
- Dried cranberries 1/4 cup
- Freshly ground salt to taste
- Pepper to taste

OPTIONAL
- Whole grain bread 4 slices

- Toppings
- Spinach
- Red onion
- Arugula

INSTRUCTIONS

- Smash the chickpeas with a fork in a small bowl, then add the avocado and smash it again until avocado looks smooth.
- Add or stir with the juice of the lemon and the cranberries. Add salt and pepper if needed. Put in the refrigerator until ready to serve
- When ready, spread 1/2 chickpea avocado salad over 1 slice of bread.
- Top with, red onion arugula, or spinach. Add a second toasted slice to the top, then cut in half and enjoy!

Walnut-Rosemary Crusted Salmon

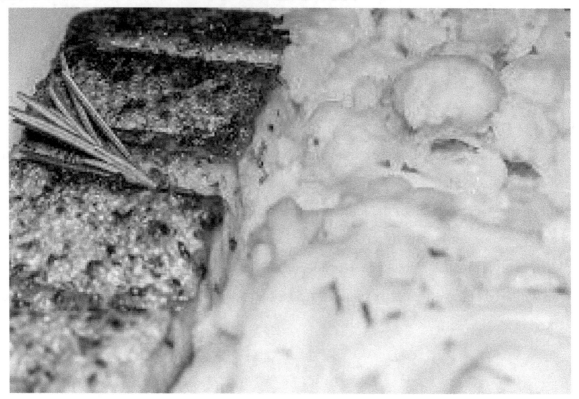

Ingredients

- Dijon mustard 2 teaspoons
- Clove garlic minced 1
- Lemon zest ¼ teaspoons
- Fresh rosemary chopped 1 teaspoon
- Honey ½ teaspoon
- Kosher salt ½ teaspoon
- Crushed red pepper ¼ teaspoon
- Panko breadcrumbs 3 tablespoons
- Finely chopped walnuts 3 tablespoons
- Extra-virgin olive oil 1 teaspoon
- Skinless salmon fillet, fresh or frozen 1 pound
- Cooking spray Olive oil

For garnish

- Lemon
- **Chopped fresh parsley**

INSTRUCTIONS

- Adjust the oven preheat 425 degrees and place a rimmed baking sheet with parchment paper
- In a small bowl combine, lemon juice, rosemary, honey, mustard, garlic, lemon zest, salt, and crushed red pepper.
- In another small bowl, add and combine walnuts and oil and Combine panko.
- Line or Add salmon on the prepared baking sheet and sprinkle with the panko mixture and place or spread the mustard mixture over the fish and coated with the cooking spray.
- Back about 10-14 minutes or until fish flakes easily with a fork sprinkle some parsley and serve with lemon if desired.

Artichoke ricotta flatbread

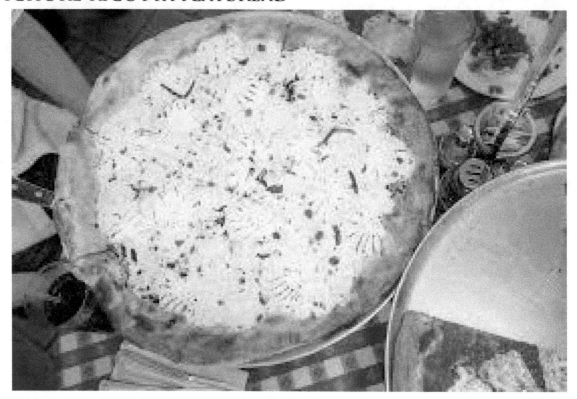

INGREDIENTS

- Pizza dough 1/2 pound
- Whole milk ricotta cheese fresh1 1/2 cups
- Fresh basil chopped 2 tablespoons
- Honey 1 tablespoon
- Marinated artichokes drained 8 ounces
- Fresh mortadella 6 ounces
- Fresh arugula 3 cups
- Fresh shaved parmesan cheese 1/2 cup
- Fresh chives chopped 1 tablespoon

For drizzling

- Olive oil
- LEMON VINAIGRETTE
- Olive oil 1/3 cup
- Lemon juice 1 tsp
- Apple cider vinegar 2 teaspoons

- Salt to taste

INSTRUCTIONS

- Adjust the oven preheat to 450 F
- Take a large baking sheet and grease with olive oil.
- Push or roll the dough out on a finely blurred surface until it is very thin. Move the dough into the ready baking sheet and sprinkle lightly with salt and potato and drizzle with olive oil. Bake, until the crust looks golden. Stir the ricotta, basil, sugar, and a pinch of salt and pepper together and remove the bread from the " Heat" when done and top with ricotta
- If desired, sprinkle with crushed red pepper flakes.
- Top with shaved parmesan and arugula and serve

Miso-Maple Salmon

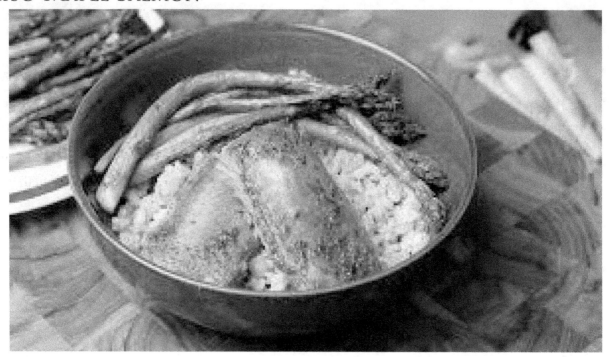

Ingredients

- Lemons 2
- Limes 2
- White miso ¼ cup
- Olive oil extra-virgin 2 tablespoons
- Maple syrup 2 tablespoons
- Ground pepper ¼ teaspoon
- Cayenne pepper to taste
- Salmon fillet skin-on 1 "2 1/2 pound."

For garnish

- Sliced scallions

Instructions

- Line a large rimmed baking sheet with foil and preheat oven to high.
- In a small bowl, add juice 1 lemon and 1 lime and combine and whisk in oil, maple syrup, cayenne, pepper, and miso.
- Add salmon, into the prepared pan and top with miso mixture.
- Add or sprinkle remaining lime and lemon around the salmon cuts sides up.

- Cook for 8-12 minutes until it flakes with a fork and serves with the lime and lemon halves if desired

Broccoli & Cauliflower Salad

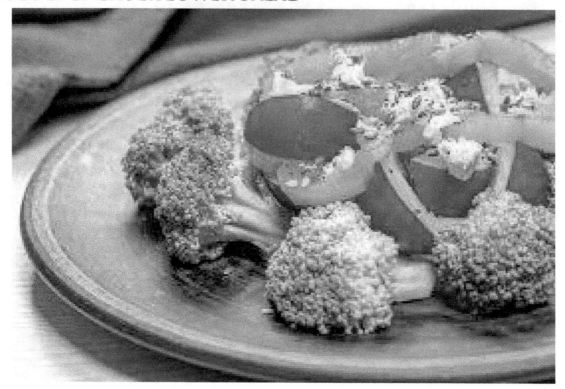

Ingredients
- Cauliflower florets 3 cups
- Broccoli florets 3 cups
- Extra-virgin olive oil 4 tablespoons
- Salt ½ teaspoon
- Ground pepper ¼ teaspoon
- Champagne vinegar 1 tablespoon
- Dijon mustard 1 ½ teaspoons
- Honey 1 teaspoon
- Chopped lacinato kale 8 cups
- Dried cherries ½ cup
- Shaved manchego cheese 1 cup
- Chopped toasted pecans ⅓ cup

Instructions
- Adjust the oven to 450 degrees and place a rimmed baking sheet into the oven
- In a large bowl, add broccoli, cauliflower, oil, salt, pepper, and toss until coat well.

- Place or spread on the baking sheet and roast about 12-14 minutes or until tender and looked golden brown
- In a large bowl, add mustard oil, honey, vinegar, and oil and whisk well Add kale for dressing.
- Add cherries and roasted vegetables, cheese, and pecans; softly toss to combine.

Roasted Beet Hummus

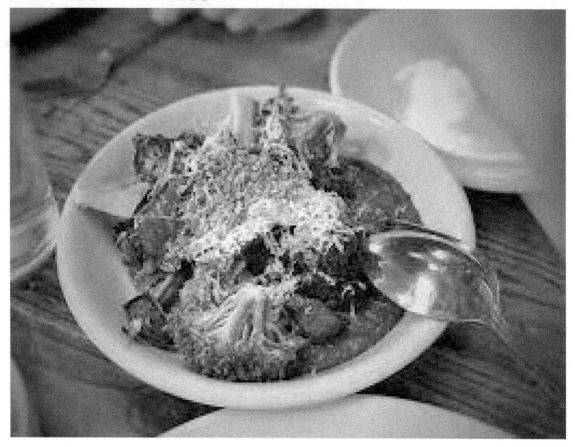

Ingredients
- Salt-added chickpeas rinsed 15 ounces 1Can
- Roasted beets, patted dry and coarsely chopped 8 ounces
- Tahini ¼ cups
- Virgin olive oil ¼ cup extra
- Lemon juice ¼ cup extra
- Lemon juice ¼ cup
- Clove garlic 1
- Ground cumin 1 teaspoon
- Salt ½ teaspoon

Instructions
- In a food processor, combine beets, tahini, oil, lemon juice, cumin, chickpeas, and salt and puree well until very smooth 3-4 minutes and served with pita chips and veggie.

Five-Spice Bacon Salad with Peach, Raspberry & Watercress

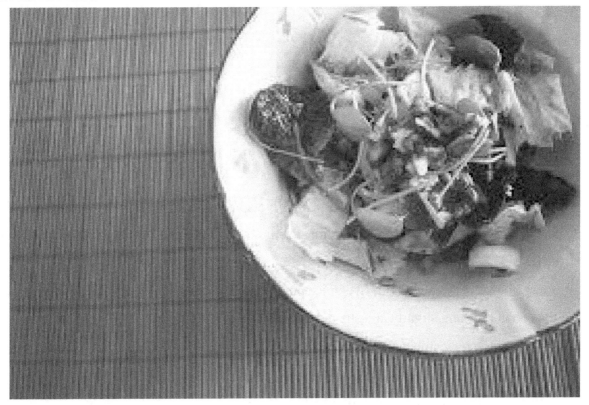

Ingredients

- Cut bacon thick 8 ounces
- Port ¼ cup
- Red wine ¼ cup
- Pure maple syrup 1 tablespoon
- Cloves garlic peeled 2
- Chinese five-spice powder 1 ½ teaspoons
- Salad
- Medium shallot, thinly sliced 1
- Extra-virgin olive oil 2 tablespoons
- Cider vinegar 2 tablespoons
- Maple syrup 1 teaspoon
- Chinese five-spice powder ¼ teaspoon
- Salt to taste
- Fresh raspberries ¾ cup

- Firm ripe peaches, cut into 1/4-inch wedges 3
- Watercress, tough stems trimmed 4 cups
- Head radicchio small ½

For garnish

- Flaky sea salt

Instruction

- Heat a large skillet and cut bacon into thick strips, then add bacon and cook 4-6 minutes or until crisp or look browned and set aside until cool.
- Add port, wine garlic cloves, maple syrup, and five-spice powder into the high heat pan until boil. Add the bacon and cook until sauce is almost completely reduced. Coating the bacon and Remove from heat
- In a large bowl, mix vinegar, oil, five-spice powder, salt, syrup, shallot, and salt and with the back of the spoon crushing slightly and stir in raspberries.
- Add watercress, radicchio, and peaches and slightly toss until coat well.
- Topped with the glazed bacon and garnish with sea salt and serve.

Beet & Goat Cheese Tartines

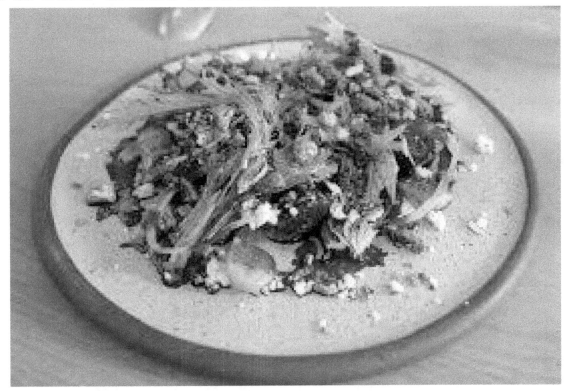

Ingredients
- Red and or golden beets 4 small
- Extra-virgin olive oil 1 tablespoon
- White balsamic vinegar 1 tablespoon
- Salt ¼ teaspoon
- Ground pepper 1 tsp
- Soft goat cheese 4 ounces
- Milk 2 tablespoons
- Crusty whole-grain bread 4 slices
- For garnish
- Fresh thyme or flaky sea salt

Instruction
- In a medium bowl mix or Stir goat cheese and milk until smooth. Season with pepper.
- Place or spread 2 tbsp of the mixture on each piece of toast and top with beets and garnish with flaky salt if desired.

- Add beets and steam, 12-16 minutes until tender.
- Set aside in a cutting board and wait for 10- minutes until cool; use a paper towel and rub off the skins, or you can use your fingers too.
- Take a sharp cutting knife and slice or wedges and cut the beets.
- Transfer this into a large bowl and slightly toss with vinegar, salt, pepper, and oil
- In a medium bowl, add milk and cheese goat and stir well until smooth, sprinkle mixture on each piece of toast.
- Garnish with flaky salt or thyme If desired

Turmeric Rice Bowl with Garam Masala Root Vegetables & Chickpeas

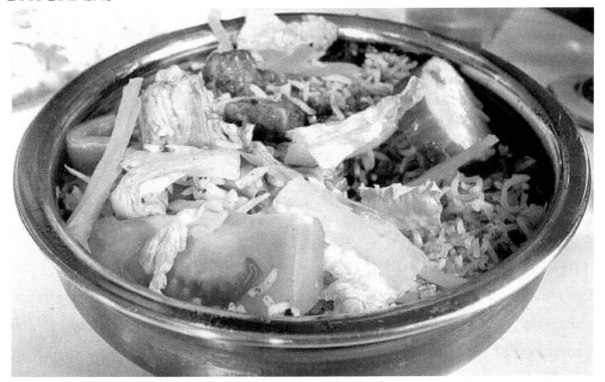

Ingredients

- Rice
- Water 1 ¼
- Brown basmati rice ½ cup
- Raisins ¼ cup
- Extra-virgin olive oil 1 teaspoon
- Garlic powder 1 teaspoon
- Freshly grated turmeric 1 teaspoon
- Ground cinnamon ¼ teaspoon
- Ground black pepper ¼ teaspoon
- Kosher salt ⅛ teaspoon
- Vegetables & Chickpeas
- Coconut oil 2 tablespoons
- Chickpeas rinsed and patted dry 15 ounce
- Garam Masala 1 teaspoon

- Roasted root vegetables 1 cup
- Honey 1 teaspoon
- Kosher salt ¼ teaspoon
- Ground pepper ¼ teaspoon
- Lemon juice 2 tablespoons
- Low-fat plain yogurt 2 tablespoons
- For garnish
- Chopped fresh herbs
- Parsley
- Cilantro

Instructions

- In a small saucepan, add and combine rice, raisins, olive oil, onion powder, cinnamon, pepper salt, and water and start to a boil and cook for 35-45 minutes until the liquid is absorbed set aside and cover for 10-12 minutes.
- Add coconut oil in a medium skillet over medium heat and add chickpeas and cook for 3-5 minutes until crispy. Pour or stir garam Masala and cook for 1- minutes until fragrant,
- Add honey or sugar, pepper, salt, and roasted root vegetables and cook for 3-5 minutes and add or stir in lemon juice
- Topped with tahini or yogurt and serve with the rice and garnish with desired herbs if needed

Roasted Root Veggies & Greens over Spiced Lentils

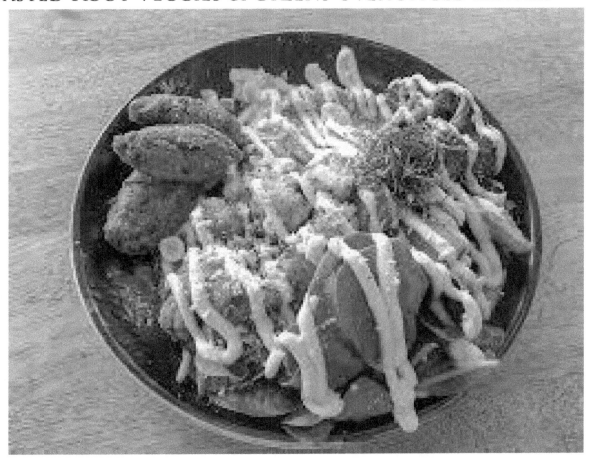

Ingredients
- Lentils
- Water 1 ½ cups
- Black beluga lentils ½ cup
- Garlic powder 1 teaspoon
- Ground coriander ½ teaspoons
- Ground cumin ½ teaspoons
- Ground allspice ¼ teaspoons
- Kosher salt ¼ teaspoon
- Lemon juice 2 tablespoons
- Extra-virgin olive oil 1 teaspoon
- Vegetables
- Extra-virgin olive oil 1 tablespoon
- Clove garlic smashed 1

- Roasted root vegetables 1 1/2 cups
- Chopped kale 2 cups
- Ground coriander 1 teaspoon
- Ground pepper ⅛ teaspoon
- Kosher salt to taste
- Low-fat plain yogurt 2 tablespoons

For garnish

- Fresh parsley

INSTRUCTIONS

- In a medium, pot adds allspice, cumin, coriander, garlic powder, lentils, water, salt, and sumac.
- Cook for 30-40 minutes until tender or liquid reduces slightly and drain and stir in oil and lemon juice.
- Add oil and heat over medium heat and add garlic in a large skillet and cook for 2-3 minutes until fragrant then added roasted vegetables for 3-5 minutes and pour or stir in kale and cook for 2-3 minutes until just wilted then mix with salt and pepper
- Serve with the vegetables and topped with yogurt or tahini if desired

Fish Tacos with Broccoli Slaw and Cumin Sour Cream

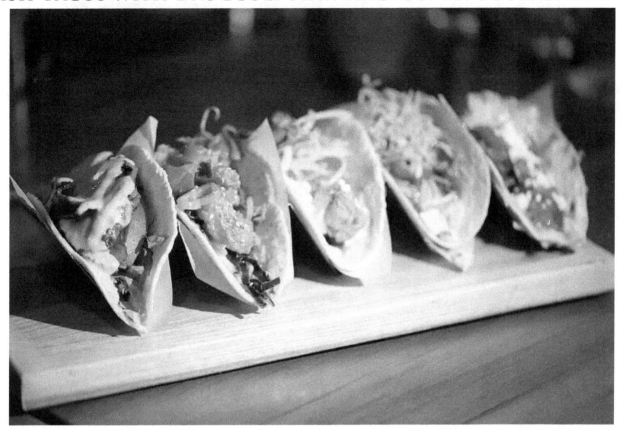

Ingredients

- Frozen fish sticks 2 10-ozs
- Broccoli 12 ounces
- Thinly sliced red onion, ½ small
- Kosher salt 1 teaspoon
- Cilantro leaves 1 cup
- Olive oil 2 tablespoons
- Sour cream ½ cup
- Ground cumin ½ teaspoon
- Flour tortillas warmed or 8 corn
- For serving
- Juice of 2 limes
- Lime wedges

INSTRUCTIONS

- According to package instructions, cook fish and divide tops from broccoli.
- With a vegetable peeler with peel stalks and cut into match sticks.
- Add lime juice, salt, and onion In a large bowl and slightly tosses to combine and set aside to marinate about 8-10 minutes.
- Slightly toss and combine stalks and broccoli oil and cilantro
- In a small bowl add sour cream, cumin and remaining salt start spread tortillas with sour cream top each taco with broccoli slaw and serve to remain and serve

Whole-Grain Cinnamon French Toast With Broiled Grapes

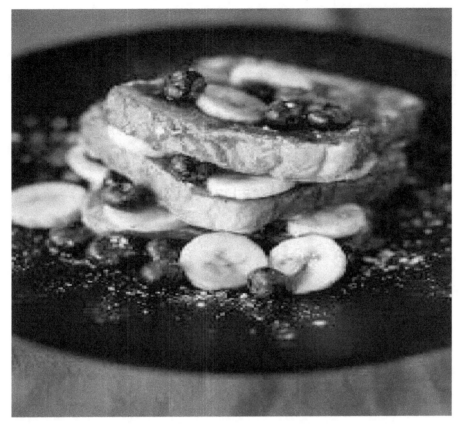

Ingredients
- Unsalted butter, 2 tablespoons
- Eggs 4
- Whole milk 1½ cups
- Vanilla 2 teaspoons
- Small loaf whole-grain bread, sliced 1 inch thick about 8 slices
- Purple grapes 1 bunch clipped into 4 portions
- Sugar 2 tablespoons
- Cinnamon 2 teaspoons
- For serving
- Maple syrup

INSTRUCTIONS

- Adjust your oven to high and lightly grease baking sheet with butter
- In a shallow bowl, add milk vanilla and eggs and beat well add bread slice into the egg mixture until dip well or centers are soaked through
- Line or place the bread slices on the greased pan and add bunches of grapes and broil for 3-5 minutes or until the bread looks golden or toasted.
- Add cinnamon and sugar and stir well until toasted.
- Set aside and sprinkle with the cinnamon sugar and serve with maple syrup and butter

Chapter Four: - Dinner Recipes

Chickpea and Vegetable Coconut Curry

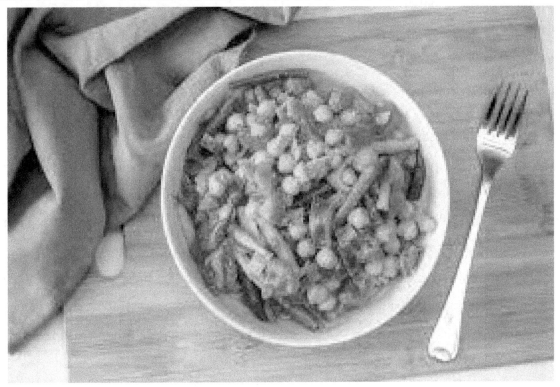

Ingredients

- Extra-virgin olive oil 1 tablespoon
- Red onion, thinly sliced 1
- Red bell pepper, thinly sliced 1
- Fresh ginger, minced 1 tablespoon
- Garlic cloves, minced 3
- Head cauliflower "small," cut into bite-size florets 1
- Chili powder 2 teaspoons
- Ground coriander 1 teaspoon
- Red curry paste 3 tablespoons
- Coconut milk 14-ounce
- Lime, halved 1
- Chickpeas One 28-ounce can
- Frozen peas 1½ cups

- Freshly ground black pepper to taste
- Kosher salt to taste
- Chopped fresh cilantro ¼ cup
- Scallions, thinly sliced 4

Optional for serving
- Steamed rice

Instructions

- Add olive oil in a medium saucepan and heat over medium heat.
- Add and Saute bell pepper, onion about 5- minutes or until tender, then add garlic and ginger and saute again for more 1- minutes until fragrant. Toss well with the cauliflower until combine. Stir in the red curry paste, coriander, chili powder, and cook for 1- a minute or until mixture looks tender and caramelized.
- Combine coconut milk and stir well with the mixture, cover the saucepan with a lid and cook for 9-12 minutes or until the cauliflower looks tender.
- Add lime juice into the curry and squeeze well until combine well then season with peas and chickpeas and season with pepper and salt.
- Garnish with scallions and cilantro if desired and serve with rice

White Turkey Chili with Avocado

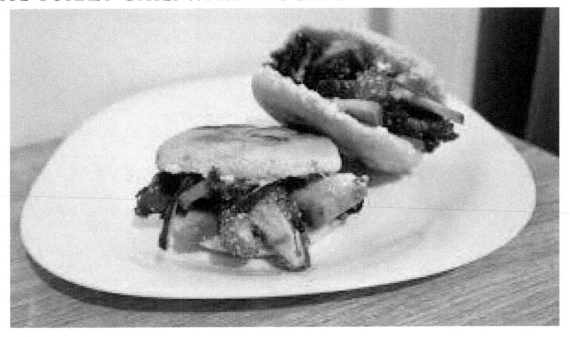

Ingredients
- Extra-virgin olive oil 2 tablespoons
- White onion, diced 1 large
- Garlic cloves, minced 4
- Ground turkey 1 pound
- Ground cumin 2 teaspoons
- Ground coriander 1 teaspoon
- Cayenne pepper 1 teaspoon
- Ground black pepper Salt and freshly
- Chicken broth 4 cups
- Corn kernels one 15-ounce can
- White beans one 15-ounce
- Avocado, diced 1

Instructions
- Add olive oil in a large pot. Add onion and saute about 6-9 minutes or until translucent then add garlic and cook until fragrant
- Dip and stir in the broth and cook the soup over medium heat for 30-35 minutes until flavors develop then mix and stir with beans and corn and simmer for more 3-4 minutes

- Add turkey and cook for 5-7 minutes until browned or fully cooked. Add cayenne, cumin, and coriander and season with pepper and salt and cook for 1-2 minutes or until fragrant
- Serve with avocado

Chicken and Snap Pea Stir-Fry

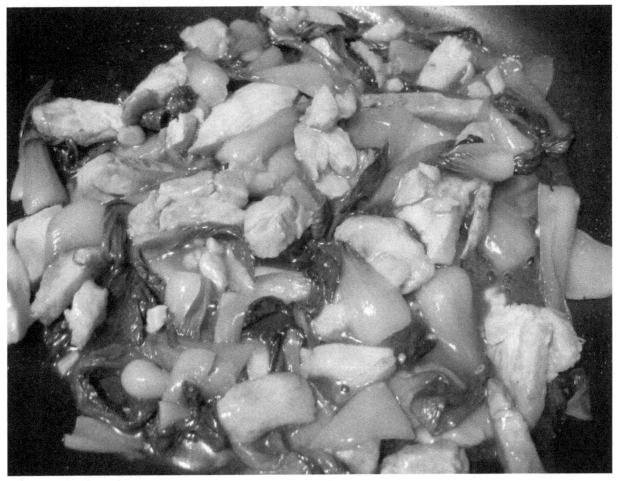

Ingredients

- Vegetable oil 2 tablespoons
- Scallions, thinly sliced 1 bunch
- Garlic cloves, minced 2
- Thinly sliced red bell pepper, 1
- Snap peas 2½ cups
- Chicken breast, thinly sliced boneless skinless 1¼ cups
- Freshly ground black pepper to taste
- Salt to taste
- Soy sauce 3 tablespoons
- Rice vinegar 2 tablespoons

(Optional)

- Sriracha 2 teaspoons

- Sesame seeds, 2 tablespoons plus more for finishing
- Chopped fresh cilantro, 3 tablespoons plus more for finishing

Instructions

- In a large saucepan add oil. Add the garlic and scallions and cook about 1- minute until fragrant. Then add the snap peas and bell pepper and cook about 2-4 minutes until tender.
- Add the vegetables and chicken and cook until golden and vegetables look tender
- Add the rice, vinegar, sriracha, and soy sauce and toss well until combine and allow the mixture to cook or simmer for 2-3 minutes.
- Garnish with sesame seeds and extra cilantro and serve

Greek Turkey Burgers

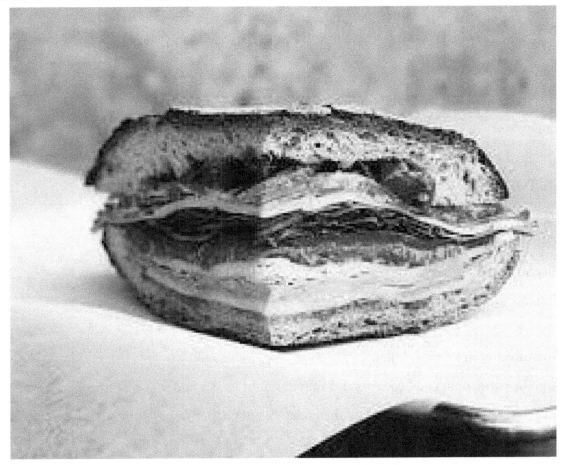

Ingredients

- Extra-virgin olive oil 1 tablespoon
- Onion, minced 1 sweet
- Garlic cloves, minced 2
- Egg 1
- Chopped fresh parsley ½ cup
- Dried oregano ½ teaspoon
- Red-pepper flakes ¼ teaspoon
- Ground turkey 1 pound
- Bread crumbs ¾ cup
- Freshly ground black pepper to taste
- Salt to taste

TZATZIKI SAUCE

- Greek yogurt 1 cup

- Cucumber, diced ½
- Extra-virgin olive oil 1 tablespoon
- Lemon juice 2 tablespoons
- Garlic powder 1 pinch
- Freshly ground black pepper
- Salt
- Chopped fresh parsley ¼ cup

BURGER TOPPINGS

- Hamburger buns whole-wheat 4
- Red onion, sliced ½
- Boston lettuce leaves 8
- Tomatoes, sliced 2

For Burgers

- Add olive oil in a small skillet.
- Add the garlic onion and cook for 3-5 minutes until tender and set aside to cool
- Mix the cooled onion mixture with the oregano, red pepper flakes, ground turkey, egg, Parsley in a medium bowl
- Season with pepper and salt and add the bread crumbs and mix until combined.
- Take meat mixture and make roll four patties of equal size and heat large oven skillet over medium heat and spray softly with nonstick cooking spray.
- Heat low and place the burger and sear for 5-6 minutes from both sides until well browned
- Move skillet to oven and cook until the burgers are fully cooked
- For sauce
- Mix, olive oil, lemon juice, garlic powder, yogurt, and cucumber in a medium bowl until combined well. Add pepper and salt and then stir with parsley
- For topping
- Add tzatziki, two lettuce leaves, two tomato slices into the bottom of the one side of burger and then place the second slice and serve

Dijon Salmon with Green Bean Pilaf

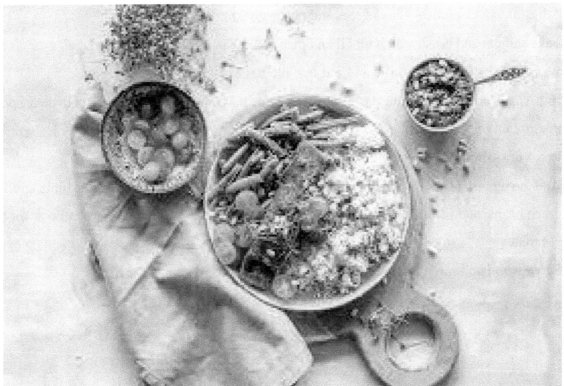

Ingredients

- Wild salmon, skinned 1 ¼ pound cut and cut into 4 portions
- Extra-virgin olive oil divided 3 tablespoons
- Minced garlic 1 tablespoon
- Salt ¾ teaspoon
- Mayonnaise 2 tablespoons
- Whole-grain mustard 2 teaspoons
- Ground pepper, divided ½ teaspoon
- Thin green beans 12 ounces cut into thirds -12
- Small lemon, zested "cut into 4 wedges" 1
- Pine nuts 2 tablespoons
- Precooked brown rice 1 8-ounce package
- Water 2- tablespoons

For garnish

- Chopped fresh parsley

INSTRUCTIONS

- Adjust the oven preheat 425 degrees and place a baking sheet with foil.
- Take salmon and brush well with oil and place on the prepared baking sheet.
- With knife or fork mash garlic and salt into the paste
- In a small bowl, add garlic paste with mustard, mayonnaise, and pepper and then spread the mixture on top of the fish.
- Roast the salmon for 6-8 minutes or until flakes easily with a fork
- Add the remaining oil in a large skillet over medium heat. Add lemon zest, pine nuts, garlic paste, green beans, and pepper and cook until beans are tender and add rice and water cook for more 2-3 minutes
- Serve with lemon wedges and bean pilaf.

Ginger Meatball Ramen with Greens and Scallions

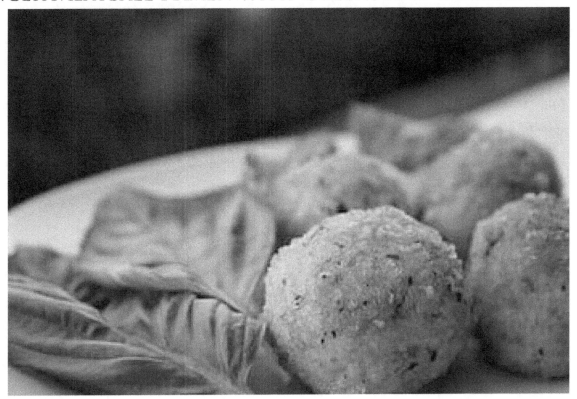

Ingredients

- Ground pork 1½ pounds
- Large eggs 2
- Freshly ground black pepper ¾ teaspoon
- Scallions, thinly sliced 4
- Grated fresh ginger 1 tablespoon
- Soy sauce 3 tablespoons
- Sesame oil 3 tablespoons
- Canola oil 2 tablespoons
- Vegetable broth 1 quart
- Mirin 2 tablespoons
- White miso ¼ cup
- Instant ramen noodles 4 3-oz. pkg
- Baby bok choy 6 heads

FOR SERVING

- Nori, cut into strips
- Add sesame oil, soy sauce, half the ginger, half the sliced scallions, eggs, pepper and pork In a medium bowl and stir well
- Add canola oil in a large pot over medium-high and cook meatballs for 8-10 minutes until browned and almost cooked and set aside and transfer to a plate
- Add remaining oil sesame oil in a pot over medium heat, then add remaining sliced ginger and scallions and cook for 1- minutes until fragrant.
- Mix or add water, broth, and remaining soy sauce and bring to simmer
- In a small bowl, add warm broth and miso and whisk well until smooth and then stir into soup.
- Add meatballs and noodles into simmer cook about 2- minutes until noodles look tender add bok choy into a simmer and cook for 2- minutes more and top each serving with scallions and nori.

Soy-Glazed Salmon Sandwiches with Watercress

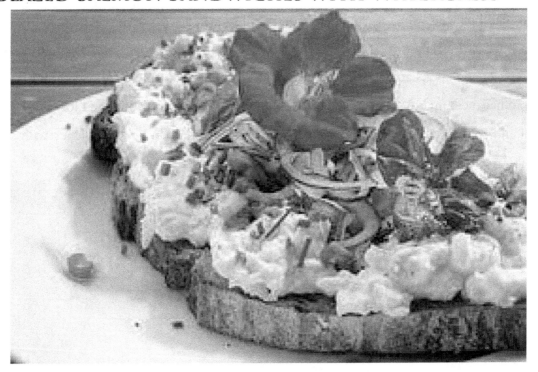

Ingredients

- Sweet chili sauce ¼ cup
- Soy sauce 2 tablespoons
- Unseasoned rice vinegar 1 tablespoon
- Canola oil divided 2 tablespoons
- Salmon fillets skinless 4 5-oz
- Kosher salt ½ teaspoon
- Freshly ground black pepper ½ teaspoon
- Watercress, tough stems removed 2 cups
- Radishes, thinly sliced 5
- Fresh lemon juice 1 tablespoon
- Mayonnaise ¼ cup
- Hamburger buns split and toasted 4

For serving

- Sweet potato chips

Instructions

- In a small bowl, add soy sauce, vinegar, and chili sauce and mix well.
- Add oil in a saucepan over medium high mix salmon with pepper and salt and cooked for 3-minutes or until looks golden from both sides and mix soy mixture and cooked for more 3- minutes
- In another medium bowl add lemon juice, radishes, watercress, and oil and toss well
- Add and spread mayonnaise on top and bottom of buns and build sandwiches with salmon and watercress mixture then served with potato chips

Mole-Spiced Black Bean and Quinoa Bowl

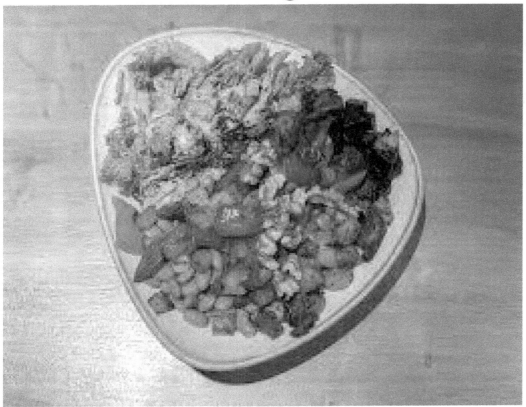

Ingredients

- Cauliflower florets 4 cups
- Ground cumin 1½ teaspoons
- Olive oil 6 tablespoons
- Kosher salt 1¼ teaspoons
- Quinoa 1½ cups
- Drained and rinsed Black beans 1 15.5-oz
- Jarred red mole sauce 6 tablespoons
- Red wine vinegar 2 tablespoons
- Honey 1 tablespoon
- Baby arugula 4 cups
- Cotija cheese ½ cup
- Roasted pumpkin seed kernels ¼ cup

For serving "optional."

- Lime wedges

INSTRUCTIONS

- Adjust oven preheat to 450 F.
- Toss cumin, oil, and salt, cauliflower on a baking sheet spread evenly into layers and roast 16-20 minutes until the cauliflower looks tender
- In a medium saucepan, add water, quinoa, and remaining salt boil over high until quinoa absorbed most of the water transfers these into a large bowl.
- In a small bowl, whisk honey, vinegar, mole, and oil mix half with quinoa mixture and add arugula and softly toss.
- Topped with pumpkin seeds and cheese and serve with lime wedges.

Vegan Green Edamame Spinach Hummus Pesto

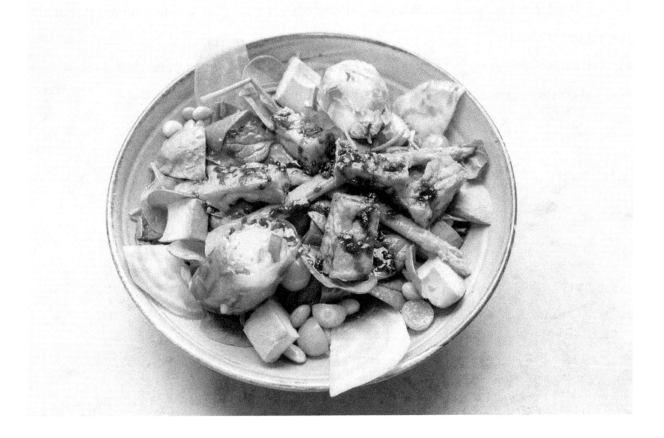

Ingredients

- Cooked edamame beans 1 3/4 cups
- Fresh spinach 7 ounces
- Tahini 1 tablespoon
- Lemon juice 1 tablespoon
- Garlic cloves, roughly chopped 2-3
- Spring onions, roughly chopped 2
- Dried oregano 1 teaspoon "or any other herb you like."
- Salt to taste
- Pepper to taste
- Optional, but highly recommended
- Nutritional yeast 2 tablespoons

INSTRUCTIONS

- In a blender or food processor and make all ingredients except the spinach and blend well until as smooth or chunky
- Add spinach and saute on medium-high heat without oil until wilted. If needed use some water,
- Fold edamame with spinach and mix and serve with pasta

Vegan Deep Dish Falafel Pizza

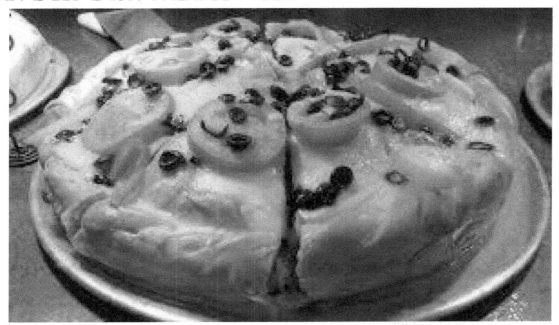

Ingredients

For the Falafel Crust:

- Cooked chickpeas 3/4 cup
- Millet, oats, or flour 1/3 cup
- Red onion 1 small
- Fresh mint 1 cup
- Fresh coriander 1 cup
- Cloves garlic 2
- Tahini 3 tablespoons
- Ground chia or flax 3 tablespoons
- Cumin 2 tablespoons
- Coriander powder 2 tablespoons
- For the Beet Hummus:
- Cooked chickpeas 1/2 cup
- Beet, boiled 1 small
- Tahini 2 tablespoons
- Cloves garlic 1
- Oregano, as desired

- Basil, as desired
- Sliced vegetables
- For the Tahini Cheese Sauce:
- Tahini 2 tablespoons
- Nutritional yeast, as desired or to taste.

INSTRUCTIONS

- Adjust the oven preheat to 390 f and line a deep pie dish with baking paper
- To Make the Base:
- In a medium food processor, combine all crust ingredients and combine well until they become little pieces. Add these on the bottom and lower side of the cake pan and spread well and bake for 20- minutes
- To Make the Beet Hummus:
- Add all ingredients in a food processor until smooth.
- Add vegetables to the hummus and mix well until falafel crust is dry then remove from the oven
- Spread and pour the beet hummus on top of the crust and return to the oven and cook for more about 40- minutes
- To Make the Cheese Sauce:
- Together with all ingredients and mix well and drizzle on top of the pizza. Serve when it has finished baking.

Chapter Five: - Snack Recipes

Turmeric Bars

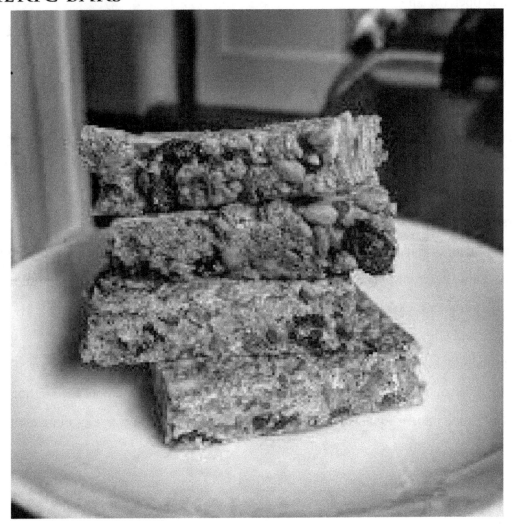

Ingredients
FOR THE CRUST

- Shredded coconut 1 cup
- Dates pitted "soak in water if hard" 10
- Coconut oil 1- tbsp
- Cinnamon 1- tsp

FOR THE FILLING

- Coconut butter 1 1/4 cup
- Coconut oil 1/2 cup

- Turmeric powder 1 1/2 tsp

For garnish
- Cinnamon 1 tsp
- Black pepper 1/8 tsp
- Honey 2 tsp

INSTRUCTIONS

- Prepare small pan and line it with foil paper or parchment paper
- Add the dates and coconut to a food processor and combine well until well incorporated, then add coconut oil and cinnamon and quickly blend. Add this mixture to the pan and press it down into pan until evenly flattened and set aside after some time place this in the fridge and chill for 2-4 hours.
- Filling a medium saucepot and Make a double boiler with water and bring it to a low boil, then add coconut Butter into the bowl and allow this to melt. Mix with coconut oil until the mixture is entirely mixed or looks like a liquid.
- Set aside and allow cooling for a few minutes.
- Stir in the black pepper, turmeric, cinnamon, and honey into the filling mixture. Spread filling over the crust and evenly spread out with a spoon then set aside and cool for 3-5 hours
- Carefully slice into 16 squares with sharp knife and top with a sprinkle of cinnamon and serve

Turmeric Gummies

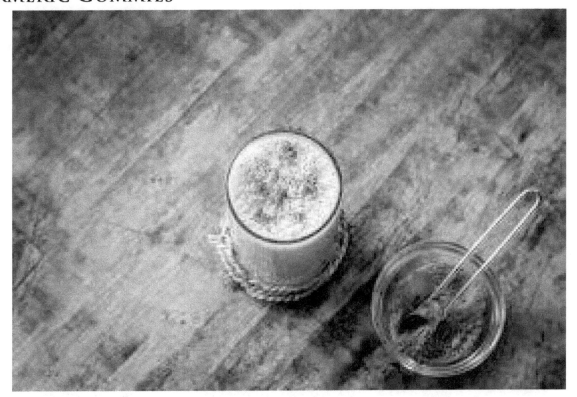

Ingredients
- Water 3 ½
- Ground turmeric 1 tsp
- Maple syrup 6- tsp
- Unflavored gelatin powder 8 tsp
- Pinch of ground pepper

Instructions
- Add maple syrup, ground turmeric, water and combine well in a large pot and heat on medium-high for about 5-6 minutes until all ingredients are well distrusted
- Remove from heat and pot and Add gelatin powder over the liquid and sprinkle well until mix well or wait until hydrate the gelatin.
- With a wooden spoon mix well and return to the heat until gelatin is completely dissolved.
- In a deep dish and pour the liquid mixture and cover it with plastic. Set aside and chill the mixture in the fridge until firm.
- slice into small squares when chilled and serve

Spicy Tuna Rolls

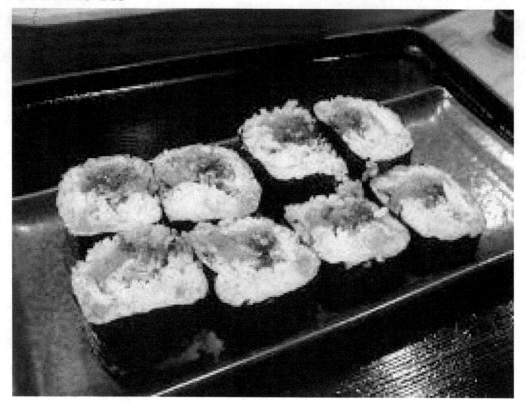

Ingredients

- Cucumber 1 medium
- Wild-Caught Yellow fin Tuna 1 pouch
- Hot sauce 1 tsp
- Salt 1/8 tsp
- Pepper 1/8 tsp
- Ground cayenne 1/16 tsp
- Avocado, diced 2 slices
- Toothpicks 12

Instructions

- Slice the cucumber lengthwise until seeds appear. Dry with a paper towel. And Set aside.
- Add hot sauce, tuna, cayenne, and salt in a medium mixing bowl and mix well until all combined.
- Spread tuna mixture across cucumber slices, one slice at a time place avocado on top of tuna and carefully roll cucumber close and secure with toothpicks and serve

Spicy Kale Chips

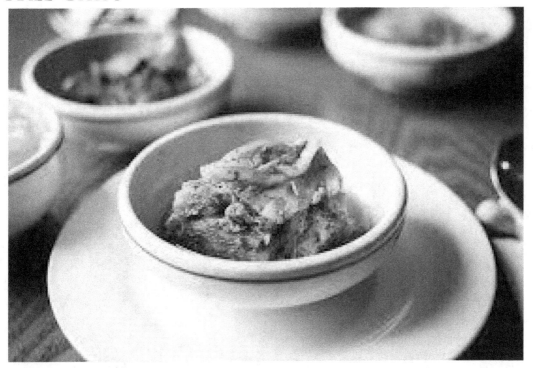

Ingredients
- Bunch of curly kale 1
- Olive oil or your favorite healthy oil
- Sea salt 1/4 tsp sea
- Cayenne pepper 1/4 tsp
- Black pepper 1/8 tsp
- Garlic powder 1/8 tsp

Instructions
- Adjust your oven to 300- F
- Dry your kale thoroughly.
- Spin dry kale in a salad spinner
- Take tear kale leaves and off their ribs into pieces on the size of potato chips.
- On a cookie sheet place, this remember to place two cooking sheets if you are making a boatload of kale it will help to cook evenly
- in your hands drizzle a little bit of oil and lightly massage it. Add or sprinkle with garlic powder, salt, and cayenne pepper to taste. And bake or cook for 15-20 minutes or until edges look crispy.

Peasy Ginger Date Bars

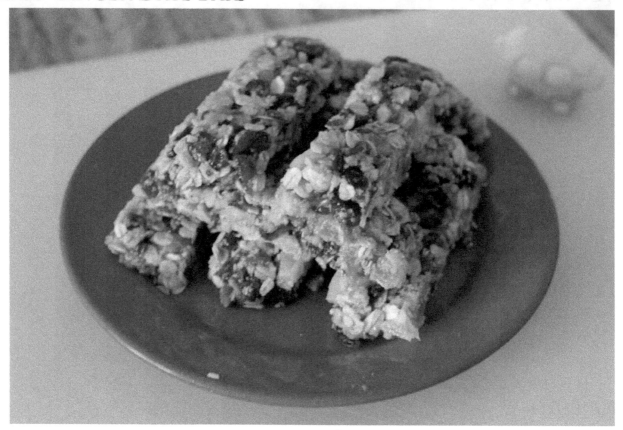

Ingredients
- Almonds 1 ½ cup
- Dates ¾ cup
- Almond milk ¼ cup
- Ground ginger 1-tsp

Instructions
- Adjust oven preheat to 350- F
- Add almonds in a high power blender and blend for 2-3 minutes or until fine and powdery. Set aside. Add dates with the almond milk in the same blender and blend for 4-6 minutes.
- Into the date mix, add ground ginger and almond flour, and blend for 3-5 minutes.
- Place or pour the mixture into a baking dish and bake for 20-25 minutes.
- Set aside until cool and slice into 6 bars.

Turmeric Coconut Flour Muffins Recipe

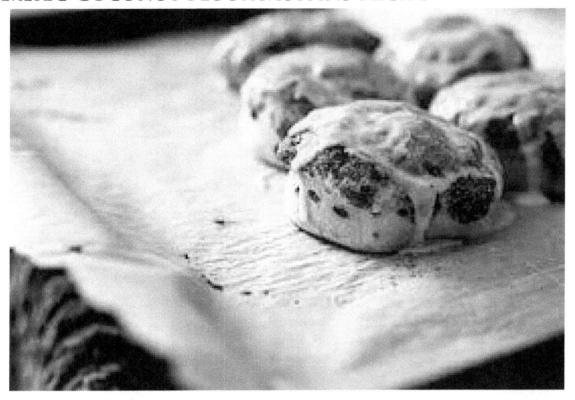

Ingredients

- Large eggs 6
- Unsweetened coconut milk ½ cup
- Maple syrup ⅓ cup
- Vanilla extracts 1 tsp
- Coconut flour ¾ cup
- Baking soda ½ tsp
- Turmeric 2 tsp
- Ginger powder 1-tsp
- Pinch of pepper and salt

Instructions

- Take 8-muffin liners and prepare a muffin tin
- Add milk, eggs, maple syrup, and vanilla extract milk in a large bowl and mix well until well combined

- Add salt, pepper, ginger powder, turmeric, baking soda, coconut flour in a small bowl. Slowly mix or stir the dry ingredients with wet ingredients until batter looks smooth and thick
- Transfer batter to a muffin tin and dividing evenly and bake for 30 minutes or until browned around the edges.
- Transfer these into a wire rack and set aside to cool and serve

Chapter Six: - Conclusion, Benefits of Anti-Inflammatory diet

We all want to grow old graciously, particularly when the risk of chronic disease is a big concern. Yet among some, pursuing the fundamentals of adequate sleep, a balanced diet, appropriate physical activity, social interaction, and stress management, which are crucial factors in sustaining good wellbeing among others, appears elusive. For example, a good nights sleep becomes vital when you are getting older, but it can be more challenging to attain. Researchers found that study participants who followed an anti-inflammation diet showed significant improvement in sleep quality. Dr. Yannakoulia and her colleagues claim that some features of this particular form of anti-inflammatory diet can significantly enhance the quality of sleep.

In another research, reports shows anti- inflammatory foods help to reduce the risk of dying from diabetes and cardiac disease. This is indeed good news.

Swedish reports suggest that the consumption of anti-inflammatory foods such as fruit and vegetables, tea and coffee, monounsaturated fats, nuts and the removal of pro-inflammatory items such as red meat, processed meat, chips and soda decreases the likelihood of mortality from any cause by 18 per cent, cardiovascular disease by 20 per cent and cancer by 13 per cent. The finding of this literature analysis was that dietary habits are linked to disease control and greater health benefits.

The anti-inflammatory diet, says Ricker, is fairly simple to monitor and can be used with better outcomes. "There has to be a nutritional change in order to be effective in decreasing inflammation."

Authors Final thought

I hope that this book has helped you discover a completely new world. It will certainly help you lose those extra pounds that you have been aching to shed-off and improve your lifestyle too.

If you wish to have quick easy, and practical cooking recipes for your healthy life, then you will refer to this book over and over again and keep it close by. After reading this book, you will be so proud of your successes when you make your tasty enjoyable meals from scratch.

I hope that you have thoroughly enjoyed reading this book and that the recipes fascinated you not in some, but many ways. Good luck with whatever you decide to do and in all your future endeavors!

God Bless always,

Rawl...